Arcady Petrov

Cosmo Psychobiology

*Improving Health
in Oncological Diseases*

Jeletzky publishing, Hamburg 2012

Jelezky publishing, Hamburg
www.jelezky-publishing.com

English 1st Edition, 06 june 2012
(1st Edition)

© 2012 English Language Version
Dimitri Eletski, Hamburg (Editor)

For further information on the contents of this book
„SVET Centre", Hamburg
www.svet-centre.eu

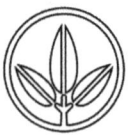

Jelezky publishing, Hamburg
www.jelezky-publishing.com

Copyright © Original Russian Language Version:
Arcady Petrov, Moscow

ISBN: 978-3-943110-45-6

© Петров А.Н., 2004
© Центр Ноосфера, 2004
© Культура

According to the responses we have received, the contents of this book have helped many people. We are confident that this will continue to be the case.

Nonetheless, we would like to point out that the techniques of Grigori Grabovoi are mental methods for the guidance of events in one's life. These methods are dependent upon one's personal spiritual development. Because we are dealing with topics relating to one's health, we give this express notice that such influence is not a "therapy" in the conventional sense of the word and is therefore not intended to limit or replace professional medical care.

When in doubt, follow the directions of your doctor or a therapist or pharmacist whom you trust! (When following conventional methods, you must expect to geconventional results.)

Jelelezky Publishing/SVET center, Hamburg

Disclaimer:

The information within this book is intended as reference material only, and not as medical or professional advice.

Information contained herein is intended to give you the tools to make informed decisions about your lifestyle. It should not be used as a substitute for any treatment that has been prescribed or recommended by your qualified doctor. Do not stop taking any medication unless advised by your qualified doctor to do otherwise. The author and publisher are not healthcare professionals, and expressly disclaim any responsibility for any adverse effects occurring as a result of the use of suggestions or information in this book. This book is offered for your own education and enjoyment only. As always, never begin a health program without first consulting a **qualified healthcare professional.** Your use of this book indicates your agreement to these terms.

Table of Contents	Page
Where does cancer come from?	5
We ourselves create the conditions in which we live!	10
How to Free Yourself from Cancer.	25
Practical Exercises	34

Cosmo Psychobiology
Improving Health in Cancerous Diseases

Where does cancer come from?

In October 2003, an excerpt from the new edition of a book by Thorwald Dethlefsen and Rüdiger Dahlke, "The Healing Power of Illness: Understanding What Your Symptoms Are Telling You" (Vega ISBN-10:1843330482) was published in the book "Harmony of Chaos" – by W.J. and T.S. Tihoplav. The following discussion is based upon the 14th chapter entitled "Cancer."

In this chapter the authors describe cancer in its inception and its development up to the point of death, the death of the cancer cell within the context of the death of its "host" human being. Cancer is described as an intelligent, but purely egotistic structure that originates out of a basically intelligent, but just as egotistical system.

A vivid description is made of all life forms and organisms, including man and his organism, as microcosms, which in turn are part of a larger, all inclusive system, the macrocosm.

Just as a person can be seen as part of a society and at the same time as an individual, who can act either conform to the society in the sense of its greater good or in an egotistical manner and against the society – against the "greater whole," the cell in the human organism can behave either beneficially or egotistically and counter-productively, destroying the "society" (the organism) to the point of disintegration or death.

The central issue is the perceived lack of freedom of the individual in society in the pursuit of his interests, which are not shaped by love, goodwill and empathy for the great common "tasks" of the cosmos, but by his egotistic, petty-minded and short-sighted thoughts and deeds:

> *"... We experience as cancer only that in us,*
> *which we also express in our lives.*
> *Our age is characterized*
> *by the heedless expansion*
> *and realization*
> *of personal interests.*
>
> *... People have cancer,*
> *because they are cancer."*

Dethlefsen and Dahlke also describe true (giving) love, the development of empathy and the vision of a greater, common unity (pars pro toto) as the only genuine remedy for cancer. And this, because – in contrast to the egotistic, cancer forming, unlived, misunderstood or perverted (selfish) "love" – it overcomes the ego and allows for openness and unity (oneness with all that is). In so doing it makes conscious, spiritual perfection possible.

The heart is the symbol of true love, for *"the heart is the only organ that is not susceptible to cancer."*

This is truly an important piece of information. One can hardly disagree with this view and there are only minor details in this chapter about which one could have a different opinion.

Nonetheless, it also happens that cancer invades the organism from the outside – in the form of a virus, an infection or information. In this case it seeks out a neutral cell, a weakened, damaged organ that is at some disadvantage. The organism inquires, "Is this something foreign to us?" This question is energetic, chemical, informational. The cancer reads the parameters of the healthy cell and docks onto it. Then it enters the cell through the receptor sites – into its nucleus – and attaches to the DNA, distorts the standard information (the well-known 25th frame effect), creates a mutation and sends the mutated cells via the cardiovascular system into the bloodstream. This is the beginning of an open battle, an Armageddon ("The Last Judgment"). In this battle the immune system usually exhausts itself. The result is that the cancer remains in the afflicted organ without supervision and continues to develop. There is no way to deal with it. It can kill immediately or in stages.

But let me make a personal remark. What is important is that it is difficult not to unite these two aspects. It is difficult to heal the person without healing his life surroundings. This also goes for the other way around [it is difficult to heal the life surroundings without healing the person], because one's life surroundings are a projection within the realm of a person's perceptions. In other words, as we think, so will our reality be. You can look at this as a process of growth beyond the consciousness of the individual person into social consciousness and back. This can also be seen as categories of indetermination that can be expressed in the concept "fuzzy logic."

For every organ, every cell, there is a mirror image in our consciousness. First comes the perception, afterwards the mirror image. And when any negative thoughts are formed in our consciousness (jealousy, hate, criminal schemes or intentions, etc.), then these create a distortion: as in the perception, so also in the mirror image. In dreams, this often comes to expression in the form of snakes, spiders, wolves and other unpleasant personifications. And our consciousness mirrors all of this again on the cellular level. Our consciousness slowly transforms into "The Kingdom of

Crooked Mirrors." It is very astounding if after a certain time some sort of pathology does not appear in the organism of such an individual, first on the energetic level and then on the somatic level.

It is also possible for such anomalies to enter in from the outside through the collective consciousness. For we are not isolated from each other and, in addition to the personal responsibility for our actions, we have a collective responsibility for what happens in the family, in society and in human social consciousness as a whole. And when within a certain circumference abnormal people with a diseased psychology, a sick imagination and unhealthy goals gather, it is not surprising that pathologies and anomalies multiply in their organism. A diseased social consciousness also makes the physical body unavoidably sick.

If you wish to live a long life and no longer be sick, then change the social life of the society and the goals it has set for itself. Dismantle the pathological, closed systems existing within the body politic and create connections to such organisms and people that strive for positive development. The cancer cells in the organism do not recognize the pronoun "WE." They know only one pronoun: "I." The pronoun I is not bad per se, but from it equal (identical) ties must be made to other pronouns. This means: I = I and, together, this equals WE. As long as this identification does not take place, what operates is: WE, that is EVERYONE, and EVERYONE = EVERYTHING.

The media hammers the thought into the collective consciousness of every person: cancer cannot be healed, AIDS cannot be healed, and so on. But in the nucleus of every cell there is a program of eternal life. But people do not know about this; no one tells them about this. Life is a closed system. In a closed system the second law of thermodynamics is indisputably at work. And when you divide the closed system into birth, life and death, you will see that behind the word "I" the word "WE" is hiding.

When consciousness is functioning correctly, then through the spirit it cooperates with the soul. And when there is misunderstanding, it seeks to extinguish the fire of the soul, a steam is created, a fog arises.

We ourselves create the conditions in which we live!

Today many people are reflecting upon how the world, how the human being is put together. And especially on the path of self-knowledge, it is justified to remind ourselves of the past. Let us cite the words of the biblical king, King Solomon, stern, even cruel words: "If you know not thyself, go thy way forth by the footsteps of the flock." In other words: Follow the path of your sheep, because the dumb and dying must follow what comes.

But when man lifts himself spiritually up to his eternal soul, diseases withdraw and he becomes the image of his Creator. For every person decides for himself, which of the two possibilities within himself he will choose, possibilities that D. Erasmus Roterodamus (of Rotterdam) so astutely discerned: "If thy body had not been added to thee, thou hadst been a celestial or godly thing. If this mind had not been grafted in thee, plainly thou hadst been a brute beast." At that time he did not know that there is also a third possibility – to connect an eternal content with the physical shell and through this connection to make it eternal as well.

Why did King Solomon say so sternly: Know yourself, or return to the path of the flock?

We enter this world to attain to experience and knowledge. We learn in order to free ourselves from a bondage that we ourselves have created because we do not perceive the world correctly. The question Jesus Christ asked every time before he began a healing of the person begging for help: "Do you believe?" was not rhetorical. It was part of a technique of freeing a person from his affliction. For the believer is already on the path to truth. In his mind he has accepted that not only can one be healed with the help of a doctor and medications, but also simply by the power of the word.

But this is only the first step. It is true that man can heal himself. Unfortunately, however, most of the people who come to us could not answer positively to the question: "Do you believe?" In their thoughts we could read something else: "I don't believe, but I hope." And still we work with such people and try to help them. And our help consists primarily of passing on the knowledge that we have received directly from the Creator. For the causes of very many diseases are similar – they are events, thoughts, actions – the things that we have done to other people, to nature, to our own or another country. We ourselves create the reality in which we live.

Why is it so important to understand and accept that psychosomatic influences form the foundation – not only of the condition of our health – but of the world as a whole? Because the world is in truth made according to the will and thought creations of the Creator. And we, his children, are created according to his example and in his image. Haven't you sometimes noticed how some passionate desire of yours was fulfilled?

Let's take a practical example. Two neighbors, the one thinks: Why don't you get sick! And the other neighbor gets sick. A layer has been formed around his life space. The relationship worsens – a crystallization forms in the communication, the "glass" phase (transparent, but hard and solid). The neighbors don't speak to each other anymore. A border has been built up between them, a wall. But talking things out is necessary. If you really communicate with each other, the wall crumbles. I am reminded of these lines from Warlam Schalamow:

"If you call forth the darkness of night, it will come. If you are jealous of your brother, so will he die."

In earlier times these words of the poet seemed to me much too conservative. But now it is clear to me that Warlam Schalamow had a feeling for underlying cosmic realities!

But now we want to continue our considerations and apply the analogies created above to oncological diseases. Cancer is a glassy, stiff reflective surface that on a deeper level produces a damaging of the tissue. If we take atoms out of the glassy reflection, the glass becomes flexible and soft. It transforms into a thin layer. You can peel it off. The layer collapses and the cells become energized. In this soft layer we enter the true information about the person's healing. Cells begin to grow and they use this layer as the basis for their growth. I repeat: first there are the cells, then the layer, which later crystallizes. We take away the crystallization and restore the layer. From the layer we produce a healthy cell.

But when such timely psychophysical effects do not appear, then in most cases the altered cell moves through the connective tissue, through the blood, through the capillary system and stops where the so-called cell drains or original cells are located. The highest energy is centered at these locations and it is exactly these areas to which the newly formed parasitic structure is attracted.

In the next stage, in the vicinity of the "drains" (they have a black color), the cumulation advances to the formation of a tumor. And in the vicinity of the "original" cells (they have a white color), the opposite is occurring; here there is an increasing loosening up of the connective tissue. Here the informational structure as well as the molecular structure of the cells that surround the damaged section is changing. After this, the cell nuclei shift and informational connections are broken. They then become tangled, which provokes the further development of the tumor.

It is necessary to diagnose the situation from the "entry" side as well as the "exit" side. The information from both sides must coincide. The entry points deliver one message – the exit points another. Between them there is a point where you can get the true information. When you focus your awareness on this information, you find access to the consciousness of the person you are examining!

Every point of entry and exit can be seen as a geometric figure. From the surfaces you can see if it is crooked or straight. A contorted geometry is a sign for deformation on the cellular level. Grigori Grabovoi has described this process very well. Geometric informational parameters can best be corrected through regular spherical shapes. Geometric informational parameters deviate from the norm in those cases where there is the destruction or loss of a supportive point in the interior of the cell.

Sign, symbol, code – this is the language of the right side of the brain: energetic forms that are bound to symbols. In order to transform an illness, you must remove its energetic form. When you take this form away from an illness, you take from it the possibility to exist parasitically in both our mind and body. And the symbol of cancer is the snake; its form on the energetic level is a fuzzy black or brown spot – the parameter of "fuzzy logic."

This is the great disaster of modern medicine: with each patient the doctors create a record of the history of disease instead of one about health. They commit untold numbers of people to disease without end. And their symbol of healing for people is the snake, which winds around the chalice of life and poisons the waters of life.

It is significant that in many countries the power of the encoding of information is perceived and made use of on a governmental level. In Great Britain, for example, signs with the warning "No Exit" were replaced with signs saying, "Exit Nearby." This is a meaningful change!

Let us repeat: space is composed of living matter. Man's environment is psychophysical and reacts to neurolinguistic encoding by the individual as well as the collective consciousness.

In this booklet you will find concrete bio-informative techniques for the improvement of one's health in oncological diseases. But let us first expand our knowledge of this little known field of science. How do we help a person in the concrete work of our own practice? Through consciousness! We do not touch anyone. We do not give any pills or shots, but the person still becomes healthy. A thought alone can save someone's life.

This is truly something worth contemplating! What separated health from disease before our psychophysical influence? Life from death? A line! This line is consciousness. Consciousness is the border and enclosure of the cell. It is the circle when it buckles and bends. The line determined the forms and became rigid. Contours arose, they became defined, and you could see that it is cancer. You have to remove these contours, the circumference, step over the line and enter into the cell. In the beginning we saw cancer developing out of the healthy cell and now we heal in the reverse order.

Man has a soul, a spirit and consciousness. But he also has good and evil within himself. He can increase the one or the other. In so doing he is not aware of what creative work means: visible and invisible matter. Man is the structure that results from the creation of form. When his consciousness reaches a certain level of development, it begins to create according to the same demiurgic laws that rule the heavens. This means it carries the demiurge ("world-creating power") of that dimension into this material dimension. And then this material dimension, which was most extremely unpleasant, turns out to hold the most promise of success. When this connection succeeds, then the so-created matter contains – in addition to the normal characteristics of man – demiurgic possibilities. In consequence, there are two possibilities: the cell can divide and spread life and, secondly, the cell can die if a person does not succeed in awakening and freeing himself from evil and a distorted consciousness.

First and Second Process:

Let us take a look at the global intentions of the Creator. Here on the Earth, the Creator created his likeness as an instrument of transformation. If you consider a person as a whole, he is the threshold between the visible and invisible. And it turns out that the invisible must still come to the fore. In general, one could say that non-material space is a scientific "research center" for the universe. Here ideas and projects are created. And on Earth we have the factory, the "workshop" in which the great ideas of the Creator are realized. The details are developed and realized by those who assist the Creator. The tools of their work are soul, spirit and consciousness.

Creative work is the prime cause of an impulse, the original source of reality that finds expression in the reaction of consciousness. Deeds of consciousness affect the soul through the spirit and inversely: the soul working through the spirit affects consciousness. The process consists of three parts and one impulse that penetrates reality and carries out step-by-step the restoration of the organism or even its revivification.

One's personal reality in the form of a reflection (a mirror image) is connected with all of reality. Such connections are constructs created by the Creator in which his power and his thought is everywhere to be found. Any construct, any connection, even those that do not even concern oneself, possesses millions of further connections, millions of variations on the theme of self-development.

In a similar manner, everything on Earth and within man repeats itself. The organism as a whole and each organ is built to serve life. Every connection that you reconstruct immediately begins to act in your daily life and in the entire world. Man can be re-enlivened. Any of his organs can be restored – in a moment. You must only consider all of the connections – within man as well as the world. These are indivisible aspects. The way in which you view man as a whole is the same way in which you must view the world as a whole.

We repeat:

"Within every cell there is structure – these are connections. Every cell is connected with other cells – these are connections. The organs are connected with entire organism – these are connections. Man is connected with the universe – these are connections!"

Let us consider how it looks with oncology if cancer were caused by information that reflects inner processes: A person has, for example, a chronic inflammation: somewhere inside, in the intestines, is the area of the inflammation. The person can live without feeling anything in particular, but in this area the environment of the cells is impaired. They are fighting relentlessly for their lives. And it is just in this mass of cells, which find themselves in such an uncomfortable condition, that in a certain moment the cunning cell-egotists appear. They invent a mechanism through which it is possible to escape from this unpleasant situation. They begin to reproduce auton-omously – they only think of themselves. They lose the receptors that regulate the speed of their reproduction. The first thing that occurs with the cells that have progressed on their way to becoming cancer cells is this: the loss of various receptors.

If you compare this process with social processes, this is the scenario of every rebellion or revolution. In the organism different organs carry out different functions. There is also dirty work to be done, for example in the intestines. But this is absolutely necessary. Without this work the entire organism would die – intestines included. But the cells of the intestines are dissatisfied with their status. They do not seek, for example, to improve the intestines through the path of developing self-perfection. They want to have everything at once – and now. Negative beings play with this dissatisfaction. They deceive the cells and enslave them. Nothing gets better by all this. To the contrary, everything just becomes worse.

Every cell has a status – the status of freedom. But this status assumes that the cell is working for the good of the whole organism. This is recorded twice in the DNA. When a cell decides that it no longer needs the status of freedom, then it erases this encoding. Most of the time this occurs under the influence of external information. Now the cell acts as it pleases. Then it really does not have any receptors anymore. It would like to change something according to its "conscience," as one says, but the cell no longer hears nor sees what is happening. It acts independently. It doesn't want to hear of God or about its responsibility. It is both deaf and blind. This is now a special species of cell, which will mutate further, because the fact that it has begun to multiply in a certain place doesn't mean it's a malignant tumor. It can also be a benign one. From the next stage onwards, it is a misfortune when this cell has the possibility to reproduce in the vicinity of completely different cells. What does this disaster normally look like? When a multiplication of cells takes place within the body, the tumor is first classified as benign, but when it begins to spread, it is classified as malignant.

In this phase of its "degradation," as a well known biologist has joked, the cell has already lost a portion of its external antennae, which receive signals, and is already in the confines of cells that are completely foreign to it. In addition, it has also lost its "professional" abilities and its sense of responsibility and declares: "I am satisfied as long as I have a blood supply. This is all I need to multiply."

Let us move from the cellular level to the macro-level – that of the external world – from the micro-scene to the social scene:

With the help of clairvoyance, it is easy to see that the core functions of the cell can continue for a thousand years! It is possible for a cell to continue to do its work for at least a thousand years! The cell is in principle a perpetual "engine," for the energy of the cell can restore itself and renew its body. Of course, one must understand that the foundation for such an immortal regime of existence can only be laid through dwelling in eternity.

Why is something else happening, something "wrong?" Why do we live for such a short and miserable time instead of for endless centuries? – Because of the false orientation of our consciousness, because of our egocentricity. People think only of themselves and try to take everything for themselves. For a short while it works. Sometimes it works for a long time when measured against the human lifespan. If people only knew what they must later pay for their striving to live only for themselves! It is easy to find an analogy. What does a person do when something in his body begins to hurt? He reflects upon how he can free himself from it. It is better when he doesn't have to go to radical measures or when the insanity of the cells that have gone crazy doesn't bring things to a lethal end.

Human egotists that only live for themselves, these are the cancer cells of the cosmic organism. Let's take a look at how one could combat these parasitic structures:

The cancer cell distinguishes itself from the healthy cells by the fact that in its nucleus the structure of its consciousness has degenerated. This means that it is thinking incorrectly, and thus it functions incorrectly. There is a saying: "He has lost his marbles."

The spiral of the DNA is wrinkled, torn. Such a cell is unfortunately not able to work creatively. It is only able to feed on what others have created. It becomes sick from egotism, something one often sees in life!

The cell only sucks up energy. In its vicinity there are also neutral cells following the motto – Not for us and not for others: an "electorate." The cancer cell uses their neutrality, pulls them in and tears the spiral of their consciousness.

What do you do in such a case? Resection, as modern medicine would do, chemotherapy? I can tell you right away: this is the path from bad to worse!

After the example of Igor Arepjev, our treatment is different. We enter into the cancer cell from which the entire situation started. The inner core of the nucleus is black and as hard as a rock. It is already unpleasant to look at the cell let alone to work with it. But this is what must be done. We reshape the spiral and remove any tears that may be there.

We destroy the information of the disease and re-enter the information of health and harmonious development. The inner layer of the cell nucleus begins to turn red, to become alive again. Already this is no longer cancer, but a benign tumor. After this step, it gets easier: two or three further corrections – and the person is healed. Hundreds of people with various types of cancer have come to us and we were able to help most of them.

Description of the Treatment:

Grigori Grabovoi works in the same manner – he instills the information that there is no cancer. He has shown us how he works. From the soul he transfers the original template or norm (the healthy state intended by the Creator) into consciousness and he reflects the information that the cancer does not exist from consciousness back into the soul. In one act the cancer is removed, in another the healthy state is brought back. For this purpose he places the number 8 (eight) over the chromosomes.

There are actually three steps to his process. He looks at the situation through consciousness (inner vision), considering all points of information. Via one point of information, he enters the informational field around the body and here he creates a movement – he removes something. Afterwards he continues in a clockwise direction: through the one point he enters into consciousness, then enters into the soul, and then enters into the tissue where the "inoperable" cancer is located. He performs a diagnosis, receives from the soul information as to the original template and moves the point where the cancer is located out to a sphere where he has for the moment (mentally) concentrated the normed information. The transformation of the structure of consciousness, its matrix, has begun. He removes the illness on the cellular level.

Another way to work is to look into the body and distinguish the diseased cells. Here we find tiny black hairs that are bent in the shape of the letter "S." On the information level such tiny hairs are symbols of cancer. These hairs take charge of the nucleus of the cell and alter it. This is when the multiplication through cell division begins.

Now, with the help of our consciousness, a new impulse is given. The patient must rebuild the structure of his consciousness. A collection of insights is created. The understanding that he is free, that he has an individual consciousness, all of this is imprinted in the matrix. This transmission is condensed into a point and enters the cancerous cell contour. Cancer is like a gluey mass that sticks to everything it touches. It is like jelly. You can't say that it is a homogeneous mass and you can't say that it is. We do not know exactly how to define it other than to call it "sticky filth."

A cancer has its own little legs and tentacles. The tentacles cut off a portion of the DNA and spray filth into the exact center of the cell. It is essential that no tentacle or part of a tentacle is left in the body. Otherwise the disease returns. This is a characteristic of the cancerous cell: if even a crumb is left behind, this crumb will multiply and continue to spread. So one needs to magnify the picture and – when you do this – you get tired! It hypnotizes the person doing the treatment. The colors change immediately, but behind the colors something is lurking!

If you return to the information level, then you see a triangle. This is consciousness. It is consciousness that adds in the colors. For example:

- A cyst is yellow, red, a watery blood color.
- Cancer is red, brown, violet, black.

Where does this effect come from? We expanded the picture and the colors changed. We saw consciousness as a very tiny triangle in a very large quadrant of space. You have to be extremely focused. It is like the headlight of a car. The light from a headlight is diffuse and not so clear for the light bulb is small. The light bulb has a reflector that disperses the light over a large area. This is an effect similar to that which one sees with cysts, with cancer and with other diseases.

Let us take a look at the optical aspect. We see colors. "What is most important here?" one wants to know. But it is really not about colors or the light bulb. The question is: What caused the disease to expand? The colors are tangential. What expanded was a part of consciousness that had concentrated itself in a point. The point then found expression in the liver, the lymph system, the gallbladder, the thyroid, the female and male organs, etc. This is an expression of the realm of consciousness… for inside the cell there are small mirrors – liquid crystals, the (computer) screens of consciousness.

Here is the connection with the organs: the realm of consciousness projects a point that goes through the thyroid and beyond. This point is a reflection of consciousness. In other words, in the realm of consciousness there is a negative point, which mirrors the problem to the thyroid and through further connections continues to mirror it. You come to the conclusion that this person harbored thoughts that were false or negative. This is primary. Color or energy – this is secondary.

How come? Because the cancer is not coming from the energy, but from a reflection of the person's consciousness. If you enter mentally into the nucleus of a cell, you see that the negative information has integrated the virus into the DNA like in the 25th frame effect and then the cancer cells multiply and multiply through the replication system of the cell, establishing themselves in some organ. After some time there follows the full narcosis and an operation.

Different people see the same triangle of consciousness differently. Some people do not see anything at all at first even when they label themselves as "psychics," "clairvoyants," or "shamans." Others see something, but via its reflection. They enter the cell and the membrane is like a mirror – on the walls there is a mirror image, a mirror image of the crystal in the nucleus. There are millions of variations on this theme.

So what do you do? If the person you are examining has an idea himself of the cause of his illness, for example, he thinks someone has put a curse on him or something like this and he even believes he knows who the person could be, then the clairvoyant, who looks into the patient's consciousness through the mirror image, sees the same thing. The opinions will be in agreement, but this will not improve the situation. The clairvoyant simply sees too many reflections, far too many. And then you have to decide which of them is central to the issue at hand. Intuition helps a bit, but the questions remain.

There is still a third variation, which works. You can create a cell according to the norm. But as soon as the cell has been created, the interconnections with the world are immediately established. You just need to create the information and it is mirrored immediately. It can be built up in a vertical or horizontal direction. If you are looking straight ahead, you see a square. If you look from the side, you see a cube.

What do you need? You have to create a point (of reference), a cell nucleus (these points then double themselves), and enter the information into this point. This is the same as when you entered the information as to the norm (of creation) into the cell for its healing. In addition, there is still the possibility of working with control functions on the informational level. This is a further variation. You go into the sphere of control. Here you immediately see mirror images, the connections with the outside world.

Within our body an unending and savage battle with viruses, bacteria and all dangerous intruders is taking place. Cancer reacts increasingly less to the standard therapies of the organism. The longest battle is the battle with oncological diseases.

The mutated cells filled with cancer information are like segments, like little hairs, from which a projection, a form is released. And this form causes an increase of the tumors. This form is carried by the blood, for example, to the liver. Here there is an entire chemical factory. Other normal cells are nowhere in sight. Why? Because here the color has changed and everything is covered over with darkness. Everything is already negatively reprogrammed. The purpose of the reprogramming is to put the organs out of commission. This is exactly what cancer does: it interrupts the course of the chemical processes in the lungs, the liver, the kidneys, the pancreas, the sex organs, the thyroid, the stomach.

How can the cancer do this? Because the consciousness of the person is distorted. Mankind is creating chemical weapons, atomic weapons – and everything that people create returns to them over a less dense, subtle level, the "scientific research center" of the universe, and mirrors itself in their organism. Who would have guessed that our consciousness is involved in this mutual exchange? However, even the weapons that are in storage are killing! They are the reflection of a certain level of the collective consciousness of man.

Cancer is intelligent! – for people are creating false inter-relationships and in our organism there exists an entire workshop that is a reflection of the external social processes. This is the real cause!

Man is a determining factor in the organization of the world. Time, space, the universe, all of this is built upon the factor "man." If man is the creator of everything, then he has the possibility of creating a wonderful life – more, he is obligated to do so. The condition is simple: "Create no filth that will then come back to destroy you."

But we are creating atomic bombs and chemical weapons. We are mean to each other instead of helping each other. All of this is mirrored and comes back to us. We create ourselves the world in which we die. We suffocate from all of this, from our malice, our hate, our polluted thoughts. We never have enough. We always want to grab something more, to manipulate someone, to deceive someone. And then everything comes back to us…

The more polluted our thoughts are, the more intelligent the cancer, AIDS and other members of the dark world.

When harmony reenters the consciousness of man, the world will become wonderful again.

How to Free Yourself from Cancer.

On the information level everything is expressed in the form of geometry, mathematics, signs, symbols, codes, forms and letters. On the energetic level cancer takes the form of a dark, fuzzy spot and on the informational level, a hexagon. The symbol for cancer is the snake. Hermes wound snakes around his staff to symbolize the power over life and death.

The snakes on the staff are the chromosomes that can be externally regulated – programs of life. When the snakes move away from the staff, it stands for the destruction of life – cancer. The form is tied to symbols. Personally, I do not like the symbol of the snake. In general, I do not like it when someone is forced to something through fear. You cannot heal the environment until you heal man. Everything here is in a mutual relationship. Can you heal through fear?

Hexagonal Form of Silicon – The whole earth consists of silicon. It forms the basis of our entire biosphere. The nucleus of the cell, the DNA, appears on the informational level in the form of a pentagon. The externality of cancer is striving to become something internal. This is a mistake. Everything has its lawful place and the attempt to take over a foreign position leads to misfortune. Man takes on the tenacious destiny: "There is no mercy to be expected from Nature." Nature begins to consider man as an infection and displaces the nucleus of man's cells with its information hexagons. In this manner the oncological processes are called forth in the organism.

Harmony! This is the key to eternal life: the appropriate behavior of man in nature and nature in man. Then man and nature will not destroy each other, but – when they work together – they will be able to reach the peak of that evolution created by the Creator. Then man can attain not only to an expanded consciousness, but also to a true consciousness – precisely that grain of sand upon which the world is built.

The various worlds will notice the truth of this, that the large is built upon the small and small is built upon the large and that the one cannot exist without the other.

Reality appears in the middle. There is a north pole and a south pole. Between them is where reality, the Earth, appears. Every creature is made in the image of the Creator. Processes of fragmentation will be replaced by the reactions of synthesis. This is happening now, in our time. So that life could be in the world, the Creator has given a particle of himself. Now that we have reached a certain level, we give ourselves back to the Creator. We become a part of him, a part of the whole.

This is reality! Although there are some who create their own reality, what they invent is a technical civilization or magic. Again another wonderland. Once you enter here, you can go for billions of years with everyone else who follows these leaders. This is not harmony. Someone is dictating what happens.

We see: an aspect of space is time, which includes the measure of space, consciousness. There is no space without consciousness, because without consciousness everything is empty. Everything exists on the basis of consciousness. The realms of consciousness are the limits of understanding. Consciousness develops itself through soul and spirit. It grows just as cells grow. They begin to breathe because of the presence of depth, height, width and circumference.

To return to our main topic, immediately after the invasion of cancer into the cell, it begins to swell, to divide, and build a second cell but with an altered nucleus and again another... And now let us look at the formation of the cancer, for example in the pancreas. Here is its tail, here its head. On the head there are many altered cells that no longer have their correct form.

It is impossible to recognize this in an early state with diagnostic devices. It does not help to carry out an operation, because the end comes very quickly – sometimes already before the operation, but more often after the operation.

Unfortunately, what we are concerned with here is a neglected stage of the disease where neither irradiation, nor chemotherapy, nor an operation has helped. What do we observe? Cells with a destroyed nucleus. When a person has undergone chemotherapy or taken oral medication, then deformations appear on the cell membrane and in the nucleus. They are immediately clearly visible. There is nothing to question here. In the cell everything is visible. This is a mutation: in the sick cell the DNA becomes visible and restructures itself.

In the mutated nucleus there are four threads in the tubulin rod (protein FtsZ). This means that such a DNA is stronger than chemotherapy or radiation. Why are these threads formed? They organize themselves under the influence of the "chemo." There comes the first chemo treatment, then the second, the third — and when the person survives, the disease changes, mutates into a new and very stable phase of its existence. And this stabilized form of cancer then begins to spread to other people, to mankind in general. It does not matter what one does, radiation, drugs, everything is useless and this is not saying enough: gruesome, when you look at it just on the somatic level.

The disease becomes resistant and threatening. This is basically the beginning of a cancer epidemic. A new form shows up in other people that consists of good, healthy cells, which are, however, subjugated to the mutations. The nucleus of these cells has already disintegrated. The DNA chain has been taken out of the nucleus and reconstructed. Or better said, the "25th frame" that you hear about so often on television is installed. And this cell will not function as expected if the area on the second DNA chain that has been destroyed is not returned to the norm.

Even when the cancer cells have been neutralized, remaining parts of them enter the bloodstream in the form of pellets or kernels. But most importantly, these kernels are what is left of the big cells. They surround themselves with microscopically small organisms. In the analyses you can see them in the blood. All of this needs to be cleaned up and this can be done by mobilizing lymphocytes from the spleen.

When these cancer cells are removed from the organism with the help of clairvoyance and psycho-physical (soul-body) influence, then it is possible to free a certain gene that moves out to the surface of the nucleus. This creates a glow and a networking with other cells. This means that it prepares this cell and others for the attack of the cancer cells. We could also introduce Magnesium or Calcium ions into the lysosomes (organelles) or prepare the unharmed cells for battle.

We observe what happens through inner vision. The gene of the cancer cell becomes visible to the outside and this cell then becomes discernable for the body's tracking system. In this case the immune system itself strangles the cancer gene in its autonomic regime. This is why it is so important to do your work early enough and not after the doctors have tried out chemotherapy, radiation, or poisonous pills.

Let us look at another aspect of this disease. When it penetrates the nucleus of the cell, it destroys the DNA chain, takes possession of a portion of it, and enters the external world through inner processes. In other words, the disease passes the boundaries of the cell, enters the organism and eventually extends past the limits of the organism itself. In this manner a person, who is restricted in his development through the disease, radiates the disease out into the external social dynamic. This shows up as accidents, ecological catastrophes, war, terrorism and other anomalies of our existence.

This leads to the conclusion: a person's disease is not necessarily just his personal affair. It touches all of us – in our personal and social consciousness. The roots of the disease lie in the past, but they are trying to grow into the future. The fruits will be bitter if the disease prevails. A healing is hardly possible if the patient is only partially healed. You must heal the whole man: kidneys and consciousness, blood and spirit, heart and soul. Nothing less.

We have been examining these issues, studying them and applying the knowledge to our practice. And we are very thankful for those who help us to unite a modern medical, conservative understanding with a new understanding, or better said, with the good but forgotten ancient knowledge. This new understanding is basically one that cannot become old because it belongs to the category of the true and eternal. At this point I would like to insert a comment. On our website we once received the message: "Doctors, oncologists, from the city of Zaparosch (Ukraine) have announced that the mechanism of the onset of cancer has an informational character." So this disease cannot only be healed through modern methods such as chemotherapy, but also with informational or "reprogramming" methods. On the one side, the wheel has already been invented. On the other, who invented it? Now we hear it from the heart of modern medicine. A praiseworthy event!

At a press conference in Kiev, the oncologist Anatolij Schugajlo announced with reference to research that one reason that cancerous tumors grow so fast is that individual cancer cells can mature and divide in as little as 18 hours, whereas the immune system of a person is set to a 24-hour cycle.

As a result of the faster cell cycle, at the time of the "inspection" of the surface of the cancer cell by the organism, the information that allows it to identify the cell as harmful has already disappeared. For this reason such cells are not destroyed and have the possibility of multiplying while at the same time they transmit the disposition for an accelerated cell cycle. A colony of such cells create the cancer tumor.

According to Anatolij Schugajlo, this finding provides the key for treatment: It is necessary to "force" the cancer cell to slow down its growth cycle to 24 hours. I must admit that this report made us very happy. It agrees with that which Igor Arepjew has seen a long time ago and with which we have been working in our practice also for a long time.

In addition, Schugajlo and his colleagues maintain that one can accomplish such an effect not only with modern medications, but also with the so-called "informational methods" of bio-energetic influence. "Some people can be healed only with the extremely harsh methods of chemotherapy, for others psychotherapy is sufficient," he says. This is a clear change from what was earlier an unshakable world view in the ranks of modern medicine! As far as chemotherapy is concerned, which actively destroys the body's immunity and contributes to the mutation of the cells, we permit ourselves to disagree with the Ukrainian oncologist. But this is a topic for a later time.

According to the opinion of Schugajlo, the differentiation of methods is determined by a varying threshold of sensitivity that is individual to different people. For this reason the doctors have chosen a combination of modern and informational methods for treatment. They have even made the public declaration: "In the practice it has been shown that informational methods significantly increase the effectiveness of taking the standard preparations." This was said by Walerij Sorokin, lecturer of the State University of the city of Zaparosch.

This discovery was made already in 1995, but the decision to make it public was reached only just recently. According to Schugajlo, there is the possibility that research on this topic will be continued in the future. But let us return to the most important statement in this report: "If one could lengthen the time to the division of the cancer cell, then the possibility of the cancer spreading would be decreased."

Truly, the less life resembles a fairy tale, the more life needs this fairy tale. But how can one use this knowledge in one's practice?

Take a melanoma (on the energetic level a dark discoloration) – one of the worst oncological diseases. How does one decode a melanoma?

In one half a minute a melanoma travels as far as a verbal expression does in a minute. The frequency or tone of the melanoma exceeds the word. In other words, it has a high reaction speed – almost double. When we enter into the double helix of the DNA, then the one helix is tight, the other is slack. In the DNA of the melanoma, the one helix is ready to break at any moment, the other is completely relaxed. Let's take a look at replacement variations.

Every molecule of the DNA also exists as a copy in reserve. The one is the working molecule; the other is the reserve. The latter is normal and gives off a normal tone. What is a tone? A tone is a resonance, an actual wave. Not too fast, not too slow, but just as it must be. So when the cancer changes the wave in the active molecule (it almost doubles the speed), you have to go to the reserve helix. The one that is active must be adjusted according to it. When there is damage in a strand of the DNA, the following happens: it locates the corresponding area on the second strand and repairs the damage according to the pattern of the copy. It perfects itself with a restoration according to the healthy template. This is called "recombination."

The DNA itself is like in a flask. Therefore, the resonance is very great. One must turn off the DNA that has been shifted by a half tone and go over to the whole tone DNA. Afterwards, with the recombination of the molecules through the informational tuning fork, that is the norm, you restore the situation to the original (active) pattern.

First you must do this in a cell and then expand the procedure. After this is done, little "pages" unfold out of the genes of the chromosomes and on them is written a text – two texts. The one text is normal ⌐ and the other, the one that is diseased, is blurred. The melanoma itself stretches out the immaculate text or tone.

We take the text from the original, normal blueprint and using this text we repair the "corrections" to the DNA that the melanoma made. This is the first step. The second is repairing the damage in the cell. In this location you find small cracks or splits. There are disturbances in the carbohydrates, the ferments and the proteins.

We take the original template (according to the norm of creation) and "push" the splits back together to remove them. "Split" had been entered into the working of the DNA.

What else do we need? We need a synthesis for what does the cell do? It synthesizes. It renews itself, reconstitutes itself. But because the process of splitting had been entered in the cell, it no longer synthesizes. Rather, it divides.

As soon as the process of synthesis begins, Death withdraws!

The repair of the working copy of the DNA and the multiplication of the cell following normal biological processes now operates according to the undamaged pattern of the reserve copy. You can distinguish between a false pattern and a correct one by the dissonant tone. If the tone has been altered by as much as a half tone, then disharmony has befallen the cell, just as in life itself.

If you cut something off from one of the ends of a tuning fork, you get a false tone when you hit it. The compressed or altered cell is like the cut off tuning fork. When in the cell, in its DNA, the lengths are different, then the resonance is also clearly different. These are the sharp and flat half tones. Is it now clear how the control system in the nucleus is constructed?

This means that the past must be corrected and the future must be constructed – so that the present moment can happen.

We have already experienced the past and made our corrections. In the future we will build up our health on the basis of the past and in the present we must maintain our health. It's as simple as this. But it seems that everyone is looking for something more complicated.

In conclusion, the slowing down of the division of the cancer cells leads unavoidably to a reduction of their growth and this signals the transition from the diseased cells to the whole tone sound. For there is a law:

"Time changes the form of everything."

And what changes time?

ETERNITY!

Practical Exercises

Every person – also those who are not (yet) clairvoyant – can work on improving their health through visualization. People, who have not yet learned our techniques, also have the possibility to help themselves and others when they use the techniques that have been especially made for beginners. Those aspects of the practical work that are for some reason at first inaccessible can become comprehensible through a process of contemplation.

One should work to increase the ability to receive information through a process of visualization (with open or closed eyes) in order to improve the results with each new application of the technique. The starting point is always the diagnosis through clairvoyance or a detailed study of the existing medical reports.

I. Performing a Diagnostic Reading:
1. Any work on the correction of a health condition should begin with a diagnosis. With clairvoyance, it is best to use red and violet colors.
2. On the beginner's level, negative information can be perceived in the form of archetypal shapes. These are the result of dark spots created in our consciousness where distorted thoughts have established themselves. And distorted thoughts project distorted forms, figures and shapes onto the screen of perception.

   A person's field of perception makes itself available through a shape or a form, or it melts together with the external information matrix. With time one develops a clear vision that is no longer dependent upon a shape.

3. You must use your direct or spiritual "power of sight." While making a diagnosis, it is important to consider why "this" has happened. (You may want to consult your intuition.) When you have found the cause, you go to the horizontal scale of time and work to change the precise event that is critical in causing the disease. Then, looking forward, see a beneficial event in the future in which you are healthy and happy.

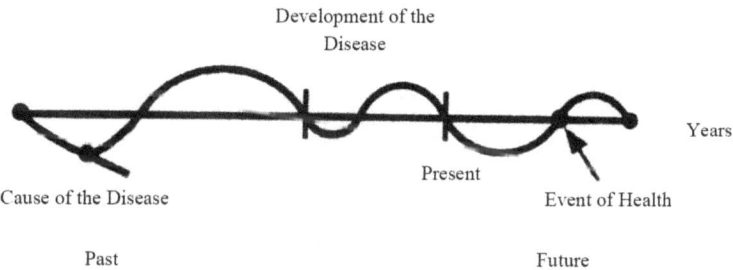

When you have completed the work on the time scale, your problem is solved to 50%. You have constructed your happy future, you have corrected the past, and you are occupied in the present with this technique.

II. Performing the Correction:
1. Once you have completed the diagnosis, you have located the area of pathology. As mentioned above, it will look like a dark spot or blotch. In this dark blotch there is a point of origin for the negative information from which the disease basically began. You have to remove this point from the organism.

   When you illuminate an unpleasant area with your consciousness such as this negative point of origin, which is hiding as dark in dark, it becomes visible through the influence of a white or silver color. The spot will try to escape your attention. Be awake and do not allow this, so that later you do not have to continually hunt it down.

Squash the spot with your consciousness and wind a silver thread around it!

Do not be afraid of it. It is not so terrible as it tries to appear. There is one thing to which you need to pay special attention. If you are only thinking of yourself, then you are – in your separate self – alone with the disease; then the disease will seem to you to be gigantic and overpowering. You seem like a dwarf and the disease like a giant. But when you consider yourself to be an essential part of the infinite cosmos, then the disease immediately becomes very small – and you very large.

Then your consciousness gains power and can squash this unhealthy spot and expel it from the organism. Direct it (mentally) to that place on the skin that is the closest. Here you will encounter a resistance. The skin is elastic and will not immediately let your prisoner out. Be insistent, stretch the pores out and press the point out through the skin. By the way, this is the same way in which the Philippine healers work that open the skin with their hands and their thoughts.

Once external to the body, the negative information loses its form and begins to disintegrate into small segments as if the scales on a snake were falling off. This happens because you have removed the form from the disease. The form of the disease had been held by your consciousness. As soon as you moved the negative point of information outside the body, it lost the mechanism of determining its form and disintegrated. This is like mixing up the letters in a game with words.

2. After you have (mentally) illuminated the area of the pathology up to the state of visualization of the cells, you have to find the first cell, the

one with which everything started. Then you enter this cell with a ray of your consciousness. You will probably see the following scene: you are standing on the bank of a river. The water is black, polluted. It is not "water of life," but "water of death." Look at it and purify it mentally until the water is clear. The verbal code for the original template is: "crystal clear water." At this point you will see the sand at the bottom of the river and various pebbles and algae. The grains of sand are liquid crystals; the rocks are organelles; the algae are receptors.

This is, of course, an allegory with which the right side of your brain presents the problem in your organism to your imagination. But this allegory is not random. It is connected with the given situation and the potential for its correction in the most direct manner possible.

In as far as the anomalies of the image were corrected, the informational situation between the left and right hemispheres of your brain is corrected as well as the informational basis of your disease.

3. Now you must exit the cell in which the information has been corrected and place yourself next to it. The first cell with which the disease began is connected with all of the other diseased cells through an information network. But now it is "normal" again. Therefore, you now give it the mental command to transform the disease information in all of the cells that it involved in the pathological change into health information. You will see how light signals begin to radiate out from this cell and how it begins to shine like the sun.

In this moment the oncological cells lose their information status. They become less dense and lighter. Many of them begin to move and to come out of the organism – to disintegrate.

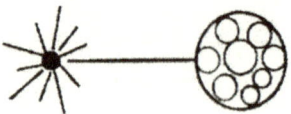

At this point a blue blotch can therefore form on the skin: a normal, blue blotch, which through the fact of its existence confirms the activity of the disintegration process. Afterwards, it becomes yellow. The most important thing to do in this moment is to direct the negative information out of the organism, to scatter it and transform it into something positive.

IMPORTANT!

The sphere from which you gave the impulse to recreate the original template should be preserved so that it has a continual, controlling influence on the situation.

There are many techniques for working with oncological diseases. This is why we advise every student at our center "Noosphera" to develop their own techniques in addition to the information that they have received here as a module, an algorithm. We would like to introduce you to a technique developed by Tatjana Bogdanowa. She is a doctor of neuro-surgery. She was first trained by Grigori Grabovoi and then at the center "Noosphera." We are bringing examples from her work, because we hope that the artistic freedom she shows will excite you:

From the information field of the ultra-distant realm of one's consciousness, one can take a living, healthy cell, a rescuer cell. We implant it into a diseased organ, where it begins to multiply.

Clockwise in the shape of a spiral, it unrolls itself and unwinds the healthy information like from a ball of twine. As it begins to increase its circumference, it displaces the diseased cells that the method described above is meant to dispel.

When you consider the fact that cancer is always seen in conjunction with an unpleasant life situation, the collapsing of the information of the life problems should be undertaken at the same time.

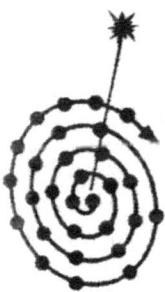

Information Expulsion

1. Imagine that we push the tumor, which has been split up into its separate cells, in between and past the muscles. We take them into the space above the head (heavenly perspective) where, on the information level, there is no skin. Each cell must be expelled through a separate cylinder and the cylinders may not touch each other. This is the model of the brain. The cells that are expelled on the information level may not cut across each other, nor may they emit any nuances of light. The light impulses must be kept under control.

Model of Non-Muscular Expulsion of Information

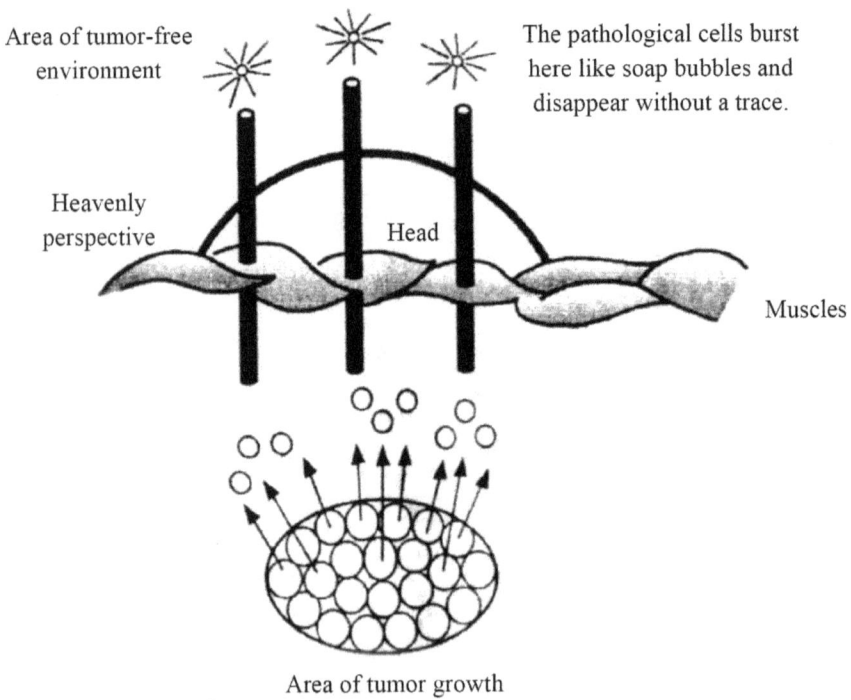

Information of the Tumor-free Environment

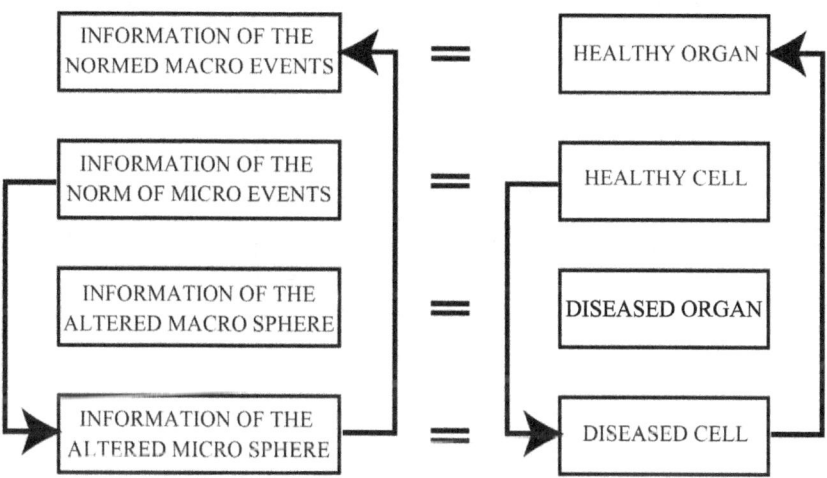

2. In the restoration process you must be able to transfer the form of the information into reality. The foundation for this work is the element of permission, allowing for this perspective to exist. The more you allow this perspective, the easier the correction to the health condition will unfold. The restoration is carried out on the basis of the phantom (on the informational level).
3. With this we conclude our instruction. We hope that you have gained much new and perhaps for you unusual information and that you are able to take what you have read and put it to work. Everything that has been given here has been tested and has proven its effectiveness.

We, as well as our students, have reached a stage where it is possible to transform negative information and energy. But especially when the destruction in the organism has gone on for a long time and was extensive, problems on the cellular level may still remain. This is the level on which modern researchers – biologists and geneticists – find their strengths.

We are not opposed to working together and hope that with time more and more specialists will connect with our work, which leads to the complete freeing of people from illness, from aging and from prostration of their creative powers. It leads to every person experiencing him or herself as a part of existence and becoming conscious of their significance for and integration with the ENTIRE COSMOS.

NOTES

NOTES

www.ingramcontent.com/pod-product-compliance
Lightning Source LLC
Chambersburg PA
CBHW051719040426
42446CB00008B/966